HERBAL REMEDIES FOR PCOS HEALTH:

"Empowering Women Through Natural Wellness"

Dr. Evelyn Stormhaven

COPYRIGHT

Contents

INTRODUCTION 5

CHAPTER ONE 10

Understanding PCOS 10

What is Polycystic Ovary Syndrome (PCOS)? 10

PCOS Symptoms and Diagnosis 10

The Impact of PCOS on Women's Health 14

CHAPTER TWO 18

The Power of Herbal Remedies 18

Introduction to Herbal Medicine 18

Traditional Herbal Practices for PCOS 22

Safety & Precautions with Herbal Remedies 25

CHAPTER THREE 30

Herbs for Hormonal Balance 30

Chasteberry (Vitex agnus-castus) 30

Saw Palmetto (Serenoa repens) 34

Black Cohosh (Cimicifuga racemosa) 37

CHAPTER FOUR 41

Herbal Allies for Insulin Sensitivity 41

Cinnamon (Cinnamomum verum) 41

Fenugreek (Trigonella foenum-graecum) 44

Bitter Melon (Momordica charantia) 47

CHAPTER FIVE 52

Herbal Solutions for Menstrual Irregularities 52

Dong Quai (Angelica sinensis) 52

White Peony (Paeonia lactiflora) 55

Raspberry Leaf (Rubus idaeus) 58

CHAPTER SIX 62

Herbs for Reducing Androgen Levels 62

Spearmint (Mentha spicata) 62

Licorice Root (Glycyrrhiza glabra) 65

Nettle Leaf (Urtica dioica) 68

CHAPTER SEVEN 72

Holistic Approaches to PCOS Management 72

Combining Herbal Remedies with Diet and Exercise .. 72

Stress Reduction Techniques 76

Mind-Body Practices for PCOS 80

CHAPTER EIGHT 84

Creating Personalized Herbal Regimens 84

Consultation with a Herbalist or Naturopath 84

Building Your Herbal Medicine Cabinet 87

Keeping a PCOS Herbal Journal 92

INTRODUCTION

In the ever-evolving world of women's health, one ailment stands as a severe obstacle, impacting millions across the globe: Polycystic Ovary Syndrome, or PCOS. This complicated hormonal condition shadows the lives of numerous women, altering everything from menstrual cycles to fertility, metabolic health, and even mental well-being. Yet, among the complications and disappointments that PCOS sometimes brings, a light of hope shines brightly: the realm of natural medicines.

Herbal treatments have been a source of healing and energy for millennia, revered by many civilizations for their inherent power and capacity to integrate body and mind. While modern medicine continues to develop, the attraction of herbal remedies has not waned; indeed, it has become more robust. As more women seek holistic methods to manage their health, the attention on herbal therapies for PCOS has grown.

This voyage into the domain of herbal therapies for PCOS is more than simply examining plants and extracts; it's an expedition through the tangled tapestry of ancient knowledge and cutting-edge research, where the lush fields of natural abundance meet the careful labs of science. It's a trip that demonstrates the incredible ability of herbs to ease PCOS symptoms, restore balance, and encourage women to take charge of their health.

Before venturing further into the field of herbal medicine, it's vital to comprehend the PCOS problem. Polycystic Ovary Syndrome is a complicated hormonal condition that affects people throughout the reproductive range. Its key features are irregular menstrual periods, cystic ovaries, and increased levels of androgens (male hormones) such as testosterone. However, PCOS is not restricted to the ovaries alone; it may be a constellation of symptoms and consequences.

- **Irregular Menstrual Cycles:** Many women with PCOS report irregular or nonexistent menstrual cycles. This may lead to issues with conception and is frequently a substantial cause of stress.
- **Hirsutism:** Excessive hair development in regions where males traditionally grow hair, such as the face, chest, and back, is a frequent sign of PCOS.
- **Acne and Oily Skin:** Elevated androgen levels may contribute to acne and overly oily skin.
- **Hair Loss:** Some women with PCOS have male-pattern baldness or hair loss.
- **Insulin Resistance:** Many patients with PCOS have insulin resistance, which may contribute to weight gain and an increased risk of type 2 diabetes.
- **Emotional and Psychological Impact:** PCOS may take an emotional toll, leading to anxiety, despair, and a lower quality of life.

The typical medical approach to PCOS care frequently incorporates birth control pills, insulin-sensitizing medicines, and fertility therapies. While these therapies may be beneficial, they may have adverse effects and limits. Here, herbal treatments enter the limelight, giving a natural and holistic alternative that complements conventional therapy or, in some situations, may even replace them.

The Herbal Renaissance: Ancient Wisdom Meets Modern Science

The emergence of herbal medicines in women's health is a more significant movement toward embracing natural healthcare. Women are increasingly seeking comprehensive solutions that respect the complex balance of their bodies. This movement is fuelled by a growing amount of research demonstrating the medicinal potential of herbs and botanicals for illnesses like PCOS.

Ancient cultures have long appreciated the healing abilities of plants. From Traditional Chinese Medicine and Ayurveda to Native American and European herbal traditions, many civilizations have used the power of herbs to treat a wide variety of health conditions, including hormone imbalances. In many respects, the rebirth of herbal treatments is a return to these time-honoured practices infused with the rigour of contemporary scientific study.

In the following pages, we will start on a riveting trip into herbal therapies for PCOS. We will investigate the herbs and botanicals that promise to reduce PCOS symptoms, restore hormonal balance, and foster the general well-being of women battling this complicated illness. From chasteberry and saw palmetto to cinnamon, fenugreek, and many more, each herb we discover has a unique tale to tell, and each has the potential to be a strong ally in the battle against PCOS.

Our excursion will expose you to the herbs themselves and the science underlying their functions. We'll dig into the science behind their potential advantages, investigating how these botanical miracles interact with the body's systems to bring about healing and comfort.

Furthermore, we will give practical information on integrating these herbal medicines into your everyday life, covering essential topics such as dosage, preparation techniques, and possible interactions with drugs or other herbs. You will find that herbal therapies for PCOS are not simply a passive addition to conventional therapy but a dynamic and proactive approach to well-being.

Empowerment Through Knowledge

At the centre of our path is empowerment. Knowledge is the key that unlocks the possibilities of natural therapies for PCOS. By studying the herbs, their qualities, and the science behind them, you can make educated choices regarding your health. You may actively participate in your PCOS management, working in harmony with your healthcare practitioner to develop a comprehensive strategy that corresponds with your individual needs and objectives.

Throughout your investigation, we urge you to stay interested and open-minded. Herbal medicines are neither a panacea nor a substitute for conventional medical care when required. Instead, they are a beneficial addition to your health repertoire, giving a natural way to symptom alleviation and overall vigour.

As we travel together into the realm of herbal therapies for PCOS, we ask you to embrace nature's great possibilities. Welcome to the herbal renaissance, where ancient knowledge meets contemporary science, hope, and holistic health bloom. Your quest for discovery starts now.

CHAPTER ONE

Understanding PCOS

What is Polycystic Ovary Syndrome (PCOS)?

Polycystic Ovary Syndrome (PCOS) is a prevalent hormonal condition that primarily affects persons with ovaries of reproductive age, often between their late teens and early 40s. A mix of numerous symptoms and hormonal abnormalities characterizes PCOS. While the specific origin of PCOS is not entirely known, it is considered to include a complex interaction of genetic, hormonal, and environmental factors.

PCOS Symptoms and Diagnosis

PCOS Symptoms:

Polycystic Ovary Syndrome (PCOS) may present in numerous ways, and not all persons with PCOS will suffer the same symptoms or with the same severity. The symptoms of PCOS might include:

1. **Irregular Menstrual Cycles:** Menstrual cycles may be rare, with missing periods or infrequent

menstruation. Some people may suffer excessive or extended menstrual bleeding.

2. **Ovulation Problems:** PCOS commonly leads to anovulation, when the ovaries do not produce eggs consistently. This may result in reproductive concerns.

3. **Hyperandrogenism:** Elevated levels of androgens (male hormones) may produce symptoms such as hirsutism (excessive hair growth on the face, chest, and other body parts), acne, and male-pattern baldness.

4. **Polycystic Ovaries:** On ultrasound, the ovaries may seem swollen and contain numerous tiny follicles. These follicles may not develop and release eggs appropriately.

5. **Weight Gain:** Many PCOS people struggle with weight control and may struggle to shed weight.

6. **Skin Issues:** PCOS may lead to skin issues, including acne and darkening of the skin in some regions, such as the neck creases, crotch, and beneath the breasts.

7. **Mood Changes:** Some persons with PCOS may suffer mood changes, despair, or anxiety.

8. **Tiredness:** Chronic tiredness or low energy levels might be connected with PCOS.

9. **Sleep disruptions:** Sleep apnea and other sleep disruptions may develop more commonly in persons with PCOS, especially in those who are overweight.

10. **Digestive Problems:** PCOS patients might have an increased risk of illnesses like irritable bowel syndrome (IBS).

It's crucial to note that not all persons with PCOS may have every symptom mentioned above. Diagnosis is often based on a combination of these symptoms and medical testing.

Diagnosis:

Diagnosing PCOS necessitates a full assessment by a healthcare expert. The following stages are often engaged in the diagnostic process:

- **Medical History:** The healthcare professional will take a complete medical history, including discussing menstruation cycles, symptoms, and family history.

- **Physical Examination:** A physical examination may involve checking for symptoms of androgen excess, such as hirsutism or acne.

- **Blood Tests:** Blood tests detect hormone levels, including androgens, insulin, and other hormones. Elevated levels of androgens and insulin resistance are frequent in PCOS.

- **Pelvic Ultrasound:** A pelvic ultrasound is used to view the ovaries. PCOS ovaries may seem swollen and contain numerous tiny follicles.

- **Exclusion of Other Disorders:** The healthcare professional will also rule out other medical disorders that might mirror PCOS symptoms.

Diagnosing PCOS is frequently based on particular criteria, such as the Rotterdam criteria, which require the presence of at least two out of three essential features: irregular or nonexistent menstrual periods, symptoms of hyperandrogenism, and polycystic ovaries on ultrasound.

Once identified, healthcare experts may work with clients to establish an individualized treatment plan that addresses their unique symptoms and concerns, including lifestyle changes, medicines, and holistic treatments, such as herbal remedies and dietary adjustments.

The Impact of PCOS on Women's Health

Polycystic Ovary Syndrome (PCOS) may substantially influence women's health, both in the near term and throughout their lifetimes. It is a complicated illness that affects several bodily systems and may lead to different health complications. Here are some of the primary ways in which PCOS may impair women's health:

1. Reproductive Health:

    - **Infertility:** One of PCOS's most prevalent and painful symptoms is infertility. Anovulation (lack of regular ovulation) may make it difficult for persons with PCOS to conceive naturally.
    - **Menstrual Irregularities:** Irregular or missing periods may damage reproductive health and suggest underlying hormonal abnormalities.

2. Metabolic Health:

    - **Insulin Resistance:** Many patients with PCOS have insulin resistance, which may lead to raised blood sugar levels and an increased risk of developing type 2 diabetes.

- **Obesity:** PCOS is commonly accompanied by weight gain and obesity, which may aggravate insulin resistance and raise the risk of metabolic problems.

3. Cardiovascular Health:

   - **Increased Cardiovascular Risk:** Women with PCOS are at an increased risk of having cardiovascular disorders, including high blood pressure, high cholesterol levels, and heart disease.

4. Endocrine Health:

   - **Hyperandrogenism:** Elevated levels of androgens (male hormones) may contribute to physical symptoms such as hirsutism (excessive hair growth), acne, and male-pattern baldness.
   - **Hormonal Imbalances:** PCOS may disturb the balance of hormones in the body, disrupting the function of the thyroid and adrenal glands possibly leading to other health complications.

5. Mental Health:

   - **Depression and Anxiety:** PCOS is connected with an increased risk of mood disorders, including depression and anxiety. The influence of PCOS on body image and self-esteem might contribute to these mental health difficulties.

6.

- **Endometrial Cancer:** Prolonged durations of anovulation may lead to an overgrowth of the uterine lining (endometrium), increasing the risk of endometrial cancer.

- **Ovarian Cysts:** While not all patients with PCOS have cysts on their ovaries, the word "polycystic" relates to the appearance of the ovaries on ultrasound.

Quality of Life:

- PCOS symptoms, such as irregular periods, hirsutism, and acne, may influence an individual's quality of life and self-esteem.

- The intensity and mix of these symptoms might vary significantly among persons with PCOS. Early diagnosis and effective therapy are critical for limiting the effects of PCOS on women's health. Treatment options often involve:

- Lifestyle adjustments (e.g., diet, exercise).

- Medicines (e.g., birth control pills, insulin-sensitizing pharmaceuticals).
- Addressing individual symptoms and concerns case-by-case.

Regular medical check-ups and consultations with healthcare professionals are necessary for monitoring and treating PCOS-related health concerns and building a comprehensive strategy to address the physical and emotional elements of living with PCOS.

CHAPTER TWO

The Power of Herbal Remedies

Introduction to Herbal Medicine

Herbal medicine, or phytotherapy or botanical medicine, is a holistic approach to healthcare that uses plants and plant-derived chemicals to promote healing, prevent sickness, and improve general well-being. This tradition has profound historical origins and is prevalent in practically every culture throughout the globe. Here is an introduction to the ideas and practices of herbal medicine:

1. Historical Significance:

Herbal medicine has been utilized for thousands of years, with evidence extending back to ancient civilizations such as the Egyptians, Greeks, Chinese, and Indigenous societies. These traditions have led to our incredible array of herbal treatments.

2. Holistic Approach:

Herbal therapy provides a holistic approach to health, including the connection of the body, mind, and spirit. It stresses addressing the under ying causes of sickness rather than merely reducing symptoms.

3. The Role of Plants:

Herbs and plants are the fundamental instruments of herbal therapy. Various components of plants, including leaves, roots, stems, flowers, and seeds, may be utilized for therapeutic reasons. These botanicals include bioactive chemicals that may have medicinal benefits.

4. Herbal Remedies:

Herbalists develop treatments from plants in different forms, such as teas, tinctures, capsules salves, and essential oils. Each state has distinct qualities and applications.

5. Traditional Knowledge:

Traditional herbal knowledge is typically handed down in certain cultures or groups through generations. Indigenous peoples, for example, have a thorough grasp of native flora and their medicinal powers.

6. Modern Herbalism:

Herbal therapy continues to develop, embracing scientific research and current knowledge of plant chemicals. This blend of ancient wisdom and current understanding is sometimes called "modern herbalism."

7. Herbal Actions:

Herbs are classed depending on their activities inside the body. Common herbal effects include:

- **Adaptogens:** Herbs that help the body adapt to stress.
- **Anti-inflammatory:** Herbs that lessen inflammation.
- **Antioxidant:** Herbs that resist oxidative stress.
- **Astringent:** Herbs that tighten and tone tissues.
- **Nervines:** Herbs that help the nervous system.
- **Diuretic:** Herbs that encourage urination and cleansing.

8. Safety and Precautions:

While herbs might have tremendous medicinal capabilities, they can also have adverse effects and interactions with pharmaceuticals. It's crucial to utilize herbs under the advice of a skilled herbalist or healthcare physician.

9. Herbalists and Practitioners:

Herbalists are those who have obtained professional training in herbal medicine. They may analyze an individual's health, propose herbal therapies, and advise on their safe and effective usage.

10. Herbal Medicine Today:

Herbal medicine is gaining popularity as people seek natural and holistic methods of health and well-being. It is commonly combined with traditional medicine to complement and improve therapy.

11. Research and Evidence:

Scientific study on herbal medicines continues, and several plants have shown medicinal promise in trials. Evidence-based herbal medicine is an emerging area that combines traditional knowledge with scient fic rigour.

Herbal medicine provides a diversified and natural approach to health and healing, anc it may be a significant component of a holistic wellness regimen. However, it's crucial to approach herbal medicines cautiously, obtaining help from certified herbalists or healthcare experts to ensure safe and effective usage.

Traditional Herbal Practices for PCOS

Traditional herbal methods for PCOS (Polycystic Ovary Syndrome) have been used in numerous cultures to address the symptoms and underlying imbalances associated with this ailment. While it's crucial to remember that herbal therapies should be utilized under the advice of a certified herbalist or healthcare practitioner, here are some traditional herbal techniques that have been studied for controlling PCOS:

1. Chasteberry (Vitex agnus-castus):

- **Traditional usage:** Chasteberry has a long history in traditional European herbal medicine. It is widely advised for regulating menstrual cycles and lowering symptoms of hormonal imbalance.
- **Potential Benefits:** Chasteberry may help regular menstrual cycles, lessen PMS symptoms, and treat specific PCOS-related symptoms, including breast soreness and acne.

2. Cinnamon (Cinnamomum verum):

- **Ancient Use:** Cinnamon has been employed in old herbal systems, including Ayurveda, for its warming and balancing effects.

- **Potential Benefits:** Cinnamon may help increase insulin sensitivity, especially for persons with PCOS who commonly have insulin resistance.

3. Gymnema (Gymnema sylvestre):

- **Traditional Use:** Gymnema is a traditional plant used in Ayurvedic medicine to promote blood sugar management.

- **Potential Benefits:** Gymnema may help increase insulin sensitivity and lower sugar cravings, which may suit patients with PCOS and insulin resistance.

4. Saw Palmetto (Serenoa repens):

- **Traditional Use:** Native American cultures previously employed saw palmetto for numerous health reasons.

- **Potential Benefits:** Saw palmetto may effectively lower hirsutism (excessive hair growth) in persons with PCOS owing to its potential anti-androgenic properties.

5. Licorice Root (Glycyrrhiza glabra):

- **Traditional Use:** Licorice root has been utilized in traditional Chinese medicine and Ayurveda for its calming effects.

- **Potential Benefits:** Licorice may help manage hormone imbalances and improve adrenal function, which may suit persons with PCOS.

6. Fenugreek (Trigonella foenum-graecum):

- **Traditional usage:** Fenugreek has a history of use in Ayurvedic and traditional Chinese medicine.

- **Potential Benefits:** Fenugreek may help regulate menstrual cycles, lower insulin resistance, and enhance glucose metabolism.

7. Dong Quai (Angelica sinensis):

- **Traditional Use:** Dong quai is commonly used in traditional Chinese medicine to promote women's health.

- **Potential Benefits:** Dong quai may help regulate menstrual cycles and decrease period discomfort in certain circumstances.

8. Spearmint (Mentha spicata):

- **Traditional Use:** Spearmint has been utilized historically for its relaxing effects.
- **Potential Benefits:** Drinking spearmint tea may help decrease hirsutism and enhance hormonal balance in patients with PCOS.

It's vital to pursue traditional herbal therapies for PCOS with caution and speak with a competent herbalist or healthcare physician. Herbal remedies should be adjusted to individual requirements since PCOS may vary widely among people. Additionally, herbal therapies should not replace conventional medical treatment but may complement it as part of a comprehensive approach to controlling PCOS. Monitoring and discussing herbal medicines with a healthcare professional is vital, particularly if you are taking pharmaceuticals or have other underlying health concerns.

Safety & Precautions with Herbal Remedies

Using herbal medicines may be a safe and effective approach to improving health and well-being. Still, exercising care and observing safety measures is necessary to ensure they are used appropriately. Here are some crucial safety rules and standards to bear in mind while utilizing herbal remedies:

1. Consult a Qualified Herbalist or Healthcare Provider:

Before initiating any herbal therapy, contact a qualified herbalist or healthcare practitioner with expertise in herbal medicine. They can help you identify the best herbs for your unique requirements and verify they are safe for you, especially if you have underlying health concerns or are taking drugs.

2. Dosage & Timing:

Always follow the suggested dose and time guidelines advised by your herbalist or on the product label. Avoid consuming more than the recommended dosage since excessive ingestion of some herbs might have severe consequences.

3. Quality and Source:

Choose high-quality herbal products from trusted vendors. Look for items tested for purity, potency, and contaminants. Herbs might vary in quality. Therefore, it's crucial to acquire them from trusted providers.

4. Allergies and Sensitivities:

Be careful of any allergies or sensitivities you may have to certain plants. If doubtful, perform a patch test or start with a tiny dosage to check for adverse responses.

5. Herb Interactions:

Some herbs may interfere with prescription drugs or other herbs you may be using. Discuss possible interactions with your healthcare professional to prevent unpleasant side effects or diminished drug efficacy.

6. Pregnancy and Breastfeeding:

Pregnant and nursing persons should take care while utilizing herbal medicines since not all herbs are healthy during these times. Consult a healthcare practitioner before taking any herbal supplements during pregnancy or breastfeeding.

7. Duration of Use:

Pay attention to the suggested length of usage for herbal therapies. Some herbs may be safe for short-term use but might have severe consequences with prolonged or excessive intake.

8. Monitoring and Evaluation:

Regularly check your Progress and talk with your healthcare professional or herbalist to assess the efficiency of the herbal therapy. Adjustments to your herbal regimen may be required depending on your reaction.

9. Side Effects and Allergic Reactions:

Be mindful of any adverse effects linked with the herbs you are taking. Common side effects may include stomach difficulties, headaches, or skin sensitivities. Get emergency medical treatment if you have severe side effects or allergic reactions (e.g., trouble breathing or swelling).

10. Storage and Expiry Dates:

Store herbal items in a cool, dry area, away from direct sunlight and dampness. Check the expiration dates on herbal remedies, and discard any that have expired.

11. Individual Variability:

Keep in mind that individual reactions to herbal medicines might vary. What works well for one individual may not be appropriate for another. Be patient and open to alterations in your herbal regimen as required.

12. Herbal Identification:

If you pick wild herbs, be utterly confident of their identification since certair plants may be deadly if mistaken for edible or therapeutic herbs. Consult field guides or a skilled herbalist for the appropriate title.

Remember that herbal medicines should not be an alternative to conventional medical therapy, particularly for severe diseases. They may complement traditional treatment as part of a holistic approach to health. Always emphasize your safety and well-being by getting counsel from healthcare experts or certified herbalists while taking herbal therapies.

CHAPTER THREE

Herbs for Hormonal Balance

Chasteberry (Vitex agnus-castus)

Preparing chaste berries (Vitex agnus-castus) for a PCOS cure entails creating an herbal tea using dried chaste berries. Here's a step-by-step tutorial on how to make and utilize pristine berry tea for treating PCOS:

Ingredients:

- 1 to 2 tablespoons of dried chaste berry (Vitex agnus-castus)
- 1 cup of boiling Water
- Honey or lemon (optional, for taste)

Equipment:

- Teacup or mug
- Tea strainer or infuser
- Kettle or kettle for boiling Water

1. Gather Your Ingredients and Equipment:

- Make sure you have all the essential materials and equipment available.

2. Measure the Chasteberry:

- Measure 1 to 2 teaspoons of dried chasteberry, depending on your liking and the intensity you wish for your tea.

3. Boil Water:

- Bring a cup of Water to a rolling boil using a kettle or a saucepan on the stove. Ensure the Water is fresh and clean.

4. Place Chasteberry in a Cup:

- Place the measured chaste berry in a teacup or mug.

5. Pour Boiling Water:

- Pour the boiling water over the chaste berry in the cup. Make sure the chaste berry is well soaked.

6. Steep the Tea:

- Cover the cup with a saucer or a tiny dish to contain the heat and scent.

- Allow the chaste berry to soak in the heated Water for 10-15 minutes. This steeping period enables the beneficial chemicals to seep into the Water.

7. Strain the Tea:

- After steeping, remove the saucer or plate and use a tea strainer or infuser to filter the chaste berry tea into another cup or a teapot. This will remove the dry herbs, leaving you with a clear tea.

8. Optional Flavoring:

- If desired, add honey or lemon to taste for flavour. Chasteberry tea may have a slightly bitter flavour, and these additions can make it more palatable.

9. Cool and Enjoy:

- Allow the tea to cool to a suitable drinking temperature. It's typically best served when it's still warm.

10. Dosage:

- Follow the suggested dose prescribed by your healthcare physician or herbalist. One cup of chasteberry tea daily, in the morning on an empty stomach, is a typical dose for PCOS.

11. Consistency:

- For herbal medicines like chasteberry to be successful, it's vital to take them regularly over time. It may take many weeks to a few months to see improvements in PCOS symptoms.

12. Monitor and Adjust:

- Regularly check your PCOS symptoms and general well-being. Consult with your healthcare practitioner to analyze the efficacy of chaste berry tea and make any necessary modifications to your regimen.

13. Be Patient:

- Remember that herbal medicines may take time to generate significant benefits. Be patient and continue taking chaste berry tea as part of your comprehensive approach to controlling PCOS.

14. Possible Side Effects:

- Chasteberry is usually regarded as harmless. However, some people may have moderate side effects. If you suffer severe adverse effects, cease usage and seek medical help.

As with any herbal medicine, it's crucial to speak with a certified healthcare physician or herbalist before using chaste berry, particularly if you have underlying health concerns or are taking pharmaceuticals. Depending on your unique requirements, They may give individualized advice on dose and use.

Saw Palmetto (Serenoa repens)

Saw Palmetto (Serenoa repens) is occasionally used as a natural therapy to help control PCOS (Polycystic Ovary Syndrome), notably to minimize hirsutism (excessive hair growth) and other symptoms connected to high androgens. It's vital to remember that although some individuals find saw palmetto beneficial, research data supporting its efficacy for PCOS is limited. Before utilizing saw palmetto or any herbal therapy for PCOS, speak with a healthcare physician or herbalist for specific counsel. If you opt to utilize saw palmetto, here's a simple tutorial on how to prepare and use it:

Ingredients and Equipment:

- Saw palmetto pills or tincture (available at health food shops or online)
- Water

Instructions:

1. Consult a Healthcare Provider or Herbalist:

- Contact a licensed healthcare physician or herbalist before utilizing saw palmetto or any herbal therapy for PCOS. They can examine your unique requirements and give specialized counsel, ensuring that Saw Palmetto is viable.

2. Choose the Form of Saw Palmetto:

- Saw palmetto is available in numerous forms, such as capsules or tinctures. Choose the format that is most convenient and acceptable for your requirements.

3. Dosage & Timing:

- Follow the recommended dose guidelines indicated on the product packaging or as your healthcare physician or herbalist suggested. The dosage might vary depending on the saw palmetto you pick.

4. Saw Palmetto Capsules:

- If you're taking saw palmetto pills, take them with a glass of Water as instructed. Follow the indicated dose.

5. Saw Palmetto Tincture:

- If you're using saw palmetto tincture, combine the appropriate dose with a small quantity of Water or juice, as advised on the product label or by your healthcare professional.

6. Be Consistent:

- Take saw palmetto continuously as instructed by your healthcare physician or herbalist. Consistency is necessary for herbal medicines to have an impact.

7. Monitor and Evaluate:

- Regularly check your PCOS symptoms and general well-being while utilizing saw palmetto. Keep note of any modifications or upgrades. Check with your healthcare professional for more information if you don't notice any favourable outcomes or encounter adverse effects.

8. Potential Side Effects:

- Saw palmetto is typically well-tolerated, although some may encounter moderate side effects, including stomach discomfort or headaches. If you suffer severe adverse effects, cease usage and seek medical help.

9. Complementary Approaches:

- Saw palmetto is commonly used in concert with other medicines or holistic techniques to address the many features of PCOS. Consult with a healthcare professional or herbalist for advice on building a thorough herbal regimen.

10. Professional Guidance:

- Regularly contact your healthcare physician or herbalist to check that saw palmetto is the best option for your PCOS treatment and has the intended benefits.

Black Cohosh (Cimicifuga racemosa)

Black cohosh (Cimicifuga racemosa) is a herb historically utilized for many health reasons, including resolving hormonal imbalances. While some may view it as a viable therapy for PCOS (Polycystic Ovary Syndrome), it's vital to approach its usage with caution and under the advice of a skilled healthcare physician or herbalist since the data supporting its usefulness for PCOS is limited. Here's some essential advice on how to prepare and utilize black cohosh if you wish to integrate it into your PCOS treatment plan:

Ingredients and Equipment:

- Black cohosh capsules, tincture, or dried herb (available through health food shops or online)
- Water

1. Consult a Healthcare Provider or Herbalist:

- Before utilizing black cohosh or any herbal therapy for PCOS, speak with a licensed healthcare physician or herbalist.

- They may examine your unique requirements, give specialized counsel, and verify that black cohosh is a good solution for you.

2. Choose the Form of Black Cohosh:

- Black cohosh is accessible in numerous forms, such as capsules, tinctures, or dried herbs.

- Choose the format that is most convenient and acceptable for your requirements.

3. Dosage & Timing:

- Follow the recommended dose guidelines indicated on the product packaging or as your healthcare physician or herbalist suggested.

- The dosage might vary according to the type of black cohosh you pick.

4. Black Cohosh Capsules:

- If you're using black cohosh capsules, take them with a glass of Water as instructed.

- Follow the indicated dose.

5. Black Cohosh Tincture:

- If you're using black cohosh tincture, combine the appropriate dose with a small quantity of Water or juice, as advised on the product label or by your healthcare professional.

6. Preparing Black Cohosh Tea (Optional):

While black cohosh is not widely used as a tea owing to its harsh flavour, some persons choose to brew it this way:

- Place 1 to 2 tablespoons of dried black cohosh root in a cup.
- Boil Water and pour it over the herb.
- Cover the cup and let it steep for around 10-15 minutes.
- Strain the tea and consume it while it's still warm.
- Note that the flavour may be intense and harsh.

7. Be Consistent:

- Take black cohosh continuously as instructed by your healthcare physician or herbalist.
- Consistency is necessary for herbal medicines to have an impact.

8. Monitor and Evaluate:

- Regularly check your PCOS symptoms and general well-being while utilizing black cohosh.

- Keep note of any modifications or upgrades.
- Check with your healthcare professional for more information if you don't notice any favourable outcomes or encounter adverse effects.

9. Potential Side Effects:

- Black cohosh is typically well-tolerated, although some may encounter moderate side effects, including stomach discomfort or headaches.
- If you suffer severe adverse effects, cease usage and seek medical help.

10. Professional Guidance:

- Regularly contact your healthcare practitioner or herbalist to confirm that black cohosh is the proper option for your PCOS treatment and has the intended benefits.

CHAPTER FOUR

Herbal Allies for Insulin Sensitivity

Cinnamon (Cinnamomum verum)

Cinnamon (Cinnamomum verum) is a regularly used spice that may give some advantages for patients with PCOS (Polycystic Ovary Syndrome), notably in regulating insulin resistance. While Cinnamon is typically safe, it's vital to cautiously include it in your PCOS treatment strategy. Here's some essential advice on how to make and utilize Cinnamon for PCOS remedy:

Ingredients and Equipment:

- Ground cinnamon (Cinnamomum verum)
- Hot Water
- Honey or lemon (optional, for taste)

Instructions:

1. Choose High-Quality Cinnamon:

- Look for high-quality ground cinnamon (Ceylon cinnamon, popularly known as "true" Cinnamon, is favoured over cassia cinnamon for its reduced coumarin level).

2. Measure the Cinnamon:

- Start with a small quantity of ground cinnamon.
- A quarter to half a teaspoon is a typical starting point, but you may alter the amount according to your tastes and tolerance.

3. Boil Water:

- Boil a cup of Water using a kettle or on the stove.
- Ensure the Water is fresh and clean.

4. Place Cinnamon in a Cup:

- Place the measured ground cinnamon in a cup.

5. Pour Boiling Water:

- Pour the boiling water over the Cinnamon into the cup. Ensure that the Cinnamon is well-soaked.

6. Stir and Let It Steep:

- Use a spoon to whisk the Cinnamon and hot Water together. This will help disperse the Cinnamon more evenly.
- Allow the Cinnamon to soak in the boiling water for 10-15 minutes. This steeping period enables the beneficial chemicals to seep into the Water.

7. Strain (Optional):

- After steeping, you may filter the tea if you like a pure beverage without the residue from the Cinnamon. However, this step is optional.

8. Optional Flavoring:

- If desired, add honey or lemon to taste for flavour. Love may also give extra sweetness to temper the spiciness of the Cinnamon.

9. Cool and Enjoy:

- Allow the cinnamon tea to cool to a comfortable sipping temperature.
- Enjoy the cinnamon tea while it's still warm.

10. Dosage:

- Start with a modest bit of Cinnamon and gradually increase it if you find it bearable.
- Consuming too much Cinnamon at once might have a strong taste and may only be suitable for some.

11. Consistency:

- For possible advantages, attempt to eat Cinnamon consistently.
- Some folks add cinnamon tea to their everyday regimen.

12. Monitor and Evaluate:

- Regularly assess your PCOS symptoms and general well-being while taking Cinnamon.
- Keep note of any modifications or upgrades. It may take some time to observe the results.

13. **Professional Guidance:**

- While Cinnamon is typically safe, it's vital to include it in your PCOS treatment plan with the advice of a healthcare physician or trained dietitian, particularly if you have underlying health concerns or are using drugs.

Fenugreek (Trigonella foenum-graecum)

Fenugreek (Trigonella foenum-graecum) is an herb extensively used in traditional medicine systems for several health advantages, including possible support in managing PCOS (Polycystic Ovary Syndrome). While fenugreek is usually considered safe, it's vital to utilize it cautiously and talk with a healthcare expert before including it in your PCOS treatment regimen. Here's a basic tutorial on how to make and use fenugreek for a PCOS remedy:

Ingredients and Equipment:

- Fenugreek seeds (Trigonella foenum-graecum)
- Hot Water
- Honey or lemon (optional, for taste)

1. Choose High-Quality Fenugreek Seeds:

- Look for entire fenugreek seeds from a trusted provider.

2. Measure the Fenugreek Seeds:

- Start with a modest amount of fenugreek seeds.

- A quarter to half a teaspoon of whole grains is a typical starting point, but depending on your tastes and tolerance, you may alter the amount.

3. Boil Water:

- Boil a cup of Water using a kettle or on the stove. Ensure the Water is fresh and clean.

4. Crush or Grind Fenugreek Seeds (Optional):

- While you may use whole fenugreek seeds, some people like to crush or ground them somewhat to release their tastes and components more efficiently.

- You may use a mortar and pestle or a spice grinder. Crushing or grinding is optional.

5. Place Fenugreek Seeds in a Cup:

- Place the measured fenugreek seeds in a cup.

6. Pour Boiling Water:

- Pour the boiling water over the fenugreek seeds in the cup. Ensure that the roots are well immersed.

7. Stir and Let It Steep:

- Use a spoon to whisk the fenugreek seeds and boiling Water together. This will help unleash their flavours.

- Allow the fenugreek seeds to soak in the boiling water for 10-15 minutes. This steeping period enables the beneficial chemicals to seep into the Water.

8. Strain (Optional):

- After steeping, you may filter the tea without the seeds if you want a transparent beverage. However, this step is optional.

9. Optional Flavoring:

- If desired, add honey or lemon to taste for flavour. Love may also give extra sweetness to counteract the somewhat harsh flavour of fenugreek.

10. Cool and Enjoy:

- Allow the fenugreek tea to cool to a suitable drinking temperature.

- Enjoy the fenugreek tea while it's still warm.

11. Dosage:

- Start with a tiny dose of fenugreek and gradually increase it if you find it comfortable. Consuming too much fenugreek at once might have a strong taste and may only be suitable for some.

12. Consistency:

- For possible advantages, strive to eat fenugreek consistently. Some folks integrate fenugreek tea into their everyday regimen.

13. Monitor and Evaluate:

- Regularly assess your PCOS symptoms and general well-being while taking fenugreek.

- Keep note of any modifications or upgrades. It may take some time to observe the results.

14. Professional Guidance:

- While fenugreek is typically safe, it's vital to include it in your PCOS treatment plan with the advice of a healthcare physician or trained dietitian, particularly if you have underlying health concerns or are using drugs.

Bitter Melon (Momordica charantia)

Bitter melon (Momordica charantia) is occasionally used as a natural medicine for controlling PCOS (Polycystic Ovary Syndrome) owing to its possible advantages in lowering blood sugar levels and boosting insulin sensitivity. If you opt to integrate bitter melon into your PCOS control strategy, here's a basic instruction on how to prepare and utilize it:

- Fresh bitter melon (available in various grocery shops and Asian markets)
- Knife
- Cutting board
- Pot or pan
- Water

1. Choose Fresh Bitter Melon:

- Select fresh, firm, and green bitter melons. Avoid those that are too ripe or have soft areas.

2. Wash and Prepare the Bitter Melon:

- Wash the bitter melon well under running Water.
- Slice off both ends of the melon.

3. Cut and Remove the Seeds (Optional):

- Depending on your desire, You may remove the seeds or leave them intact. The seeds are edible but add to the bitterness of the fruit.

- If you want to remove the seeds, cut the bitter melon lengthwise, and then use a spoon to scoop out the seeds and any pith.

4. Slice or Dice the Bitter Melon:

- Slice or cut the prepared bitter melon into pieces of your chosen size. The pieces' size depends on how you want to prepare or eat them.

5. Cooking Methods:

- Bitter melon may be cooked in numerous ways, including stir-frying, sautéing, or adding it to soups and stews. Here's a primary stir-frying method:
- ✓ Heat a saucepan or skillet over medium heat and add a small quantity of oil (e.g., olive or vegetable).
- ✓ Add the sliced or diced bitter melon to the hot oil.
- ✓ Stir-fry the bitter melon for several minutes until it becomes soft and slightly crunchy, stirring regularly. To taste, you may season it with salt, pepper, or other spices.

6. Serve and Enjoy:

- Please remove it from the fire once the bitter melon is cooked to your taste.
- Serve it as a side dish or as a more extensive dinner.

7. Dosage and Consistency:

- The amount and frequency of bitter melon eating might vary depending on individual tastes and tolerance. Some individuals drink bitter melon routinely as part of their diet, while others use it sporadically.

8. Monitor and Evaluate:

- Regularly check your PCOS symptoms and general well-being while integrating bitter melon into your diet. Keep note of any modifications or improvements over time.

9. Professional Guidance:

- While bitter melon is usually considered safe, it's vital to include it in your PCOS treatment plan with the advice of a healthcare physician or trained dietitian, particularly if you have underlying health concerns or are using drugs.

Bitter melon may be an acquired taste owing to its bitterness, but it can be savoured when appropriately cooked and integrated into many meals. It is often used as part of a balanced diet with other dietary and lifestyle adjustments as part of a comprehensive approach to addressing PCOS. Always emphasize your safety and well-being by getting counsel from experienced healthcare experts when utilizing plants or foods as cures.

CHAPTER FIVE

Herbal Solutions for Menstrual Irregularities

Dong Quai (Angelica sinensis)

Dong Quai (Angelica sinensis), often known as female ginseng, is a herb long utilized in Chinese medicine to treat different health conditions, including hormone abnormalities. While it is occasionally explored for PCOS (Polycystic Ovary Syndrome), its usage should be cautiously and under the advice of a skilled healthcare physician or herbalist since research data supporting its usefulness for PCOS is minimal. If you opt to utilize Dong Quai as part of your PCOS treatment strategy, here's some essential advice on how to prepare and use it:

Ingredients and Equipment:

- Dong Quai root (available in dried form or as a tincture)
- Water (for preparing tea)
- Honey or lemon (optional, for taste)

1. Choose High-Quality Dong Quai:

- Look for high-quality Dong Quai root from a recognized supplier. You may get it in dried form or as a tincture.

2. Measure the Dong Quai:

- If using dried Dong Quai root, start with a small quantity, 1 to 2 tablespoons of dry root per cup of tea. You may modify the amount depending on your tastes and tolerance.

- If using a tincture, follow the suggested dose guidelines indicated on the product label or as instructed by your healthcare physician or herbalist.

3. Boil Water:

- Boil a cup of Water using a kettle or on the stove. Ensure the Water is fresh and clean.

4. Preparing Dong Quai Tea:

- Place the measured dried Dong Quai root in a cup.

5. Pour Boiling Water:

- Pour the boiling water over the Dong Quai root in the cup. Ensure that the plant is well immersed.

6. Stir and Let It Steep:

- Use a spoon to mix the Dong Quai root and boiling Water together.

- Allow the Dong Quai root to soak in the heated Water for 10-15 minutes. This steeping period enables the beneficial chemicals to seep into the Water.

7. Strain (Optional):

- After steeping, you may filter the tea without the herb if you want a transparent beverage. However, this step is optional.

8. Optional Flavoring:

- If desired, add honey or lemon to taste for flavour. These ingredients help hide the relatively harsh flavour of Dong Quai.

9. Cool and Enjoy:

- Allow the Dong Quai tea to cool to a suitable drinking temperature.
- Enjoy the Dong Quai tea while it's still warm.

10. Dosage:

- Follow the suggested dose supplied by your healthcare physician herbalist or, as mentioned on the product label, if you use a tincture.

11. Consistency:

- For possible advantages, seek to eat Dong Quai regularly as instructed by your healthcare physician or herbalist. Consistency is necessary for herbal medicines to have an impact.

12. Monitor and Evaluate:

- Regularly check your PCOS symptoms and general well-being while utilizing Dong Quai. Keep note of any modifications or upgrades. It may take some time to observe the results.

13. Professional Guidance:

- While Dong Quai is usually regarded as safe, it's vital to include it in your PCOS treatment strategy under the advice of a healthcare physician or herbalist, particularly if you have underlying health concerns or are using drugs.

White Peony (Paeonia lactiflora)

White peony (Paeonia lactiflora) is a plant extensively used in traditional Chinese medicine for many health conditions, including hormonal abnormalit es. Some persons with PCOS (Polycystic Ovary Syndrome) consider utilizing white peony as part of their treatment strategy. However, its usage should be done carefully and under the advice of a skilled healthcare physician or herbalist. Here's a basic tutorial on how to prepare and utilize white peony for a PCOS remedy:

Ingredients and Equipment:

- White peony root (available in dried form or as a tincture)
- Water (for preparing tea)
- Honey or lemon (optional, for taste)

Instructions:

1. Choose High-Quality White Peony Root:

- Look for high-quality white peony roots from a reliable supplier. You may get it in dried form or as a tincture.

2. Measure the White Peony Root:

- Start with a small quantity of dried white peony root, such as 1 to 2 tablespoons of dry root per cup of tea. You may modify the amount depending on your tastes and tolerance.
- If using a tincture, follow the suggested dose guidelines indicated on the product label or as instructed by your healthcare physician or herbalist.

3. Boil Water:

- Boil a cup of Water using a kettle or on the stove. Ensure the Water is fresh and clean.

4. Preparing White Peony Tea:

- Place the measured dried white peony root in a cup.

5. Pour Boiling Water:

- Pour the boiling water over the white peony root in the cup. Ensure that the heart is thoroughly immersed.

6. Stir and Let It Steep:

- Use a spoon to whisk the white peony root and boiling Water together.

- Allow the white peony root to soak in the boiling water for 10-15 minutes. This steeping period enables the beneficial chemicals to seep into the Water.

7. Strain (Optional):

- After steeping, you may filter the tea without the root if you want a clear drink. However, this step is optional.

8. Optional Flavoring:

- If desired, add honey or lemon to taste for flavour. These ingredients enhance the flavour of the tea.

9. Cool and Enjoy:

- Allow the white peony tea to cool to a comfortable drinking temperature.

- Enjoy the white peony tea while it's still warm.

10. Dosage:

- Follow the suggested dose supplied by your healthcare physician herbalist or as mentioned on the product label if you use a tincture.

11. Consistency:

- For possible advantages, attempt to eat white peonies regularly as instructed by your healthcare physician or herbalist. Consistency is necessary for herbal medicines to have an impact.

12. Monitor and Evaluate:

- Regularly check your PCOS symptoms and general well-being while utilizing white peony. Keep note of any modifications or upgrades. It may take some time to observe the results.

13. Professional Guidance:

- While white peony is usually considered safe, it's vital to include it in your PCOS treatment plan with the advice of a healthcare physician or herbalist, particularly if you have underlying health concerns or are using drugs.

Raspberry Leaf (Rubus idaeus)

Raspberry leaf (Rubus idaeus) is a plant noted for its possible health advantages, including uterine toning and hormonal balancing. Some persons with PCOS (Polycystic

Ovary Syndrome) consider utilizing raspberry leaf as part of their comprehensive care approach. While scientific data supporting its usefulness for PCOS is minimal, it may be taken carefully by a skilled healthcare physician or herbalist. Here's a basic tutorial on how to prepare and utilize raspberry leaves for a PCOS remedy:

Ingredients and Equipment:

- Dried raspberry leaves (available in loose-leaf form or as tea bags)
- Water Honey or lemon (optional, for taste)

Instructions:

1. Choose High-Quality Raspberry Leaves:

- Look for high-quality dried raspberry leaves from a reliable vendor. You may get them in loose-leaf form or as pre-packaged tea bags.

2. Measure Raspberry Leaves:

- If using loose-leaf raspberry leaves, start with 1 to 2 tablespoons of dried leaves per cup of tea. You may modify the amount depending on your tastes and tolerance.
- If using tea bags, follow the suggested serving size on the label.

3. Boil Water:

- Boil a cup of Water using a kettle or on the stove. Ensure the Water is fresh and clean.

4. Preparing Raspberry Leaf Tea:

- Place the measured dried raspberry leaves in a cup.

5. Pour Boiling Water:

- Pour the boiling water over the raspberry leaves into the cup. Ensure that the leaves are thoroughly immersed.

6. Stir and Let It Steep:

- Use a spoon to whisk the raspberry leaves and boiling Water together.
- Allow the raspberry leaves to soak in the boiling water for 5-10 minutes. This steeping period enables the beneficial chemicals to seep into the Water.

7. Strain (Optional):

- After steeping, you may filter the tea without the leaves if you like a transparent beverage. However, this step is optional.

8. Optional Flavoring:

- If desired, add honey or lemon to taste for flavour. These ingredients improve the flavour of the tea.

9. Cool and Enjoy:

- Allow the raspberry leaf tea to cool to a suitable sipping temperature.
- Enjoy the raspberry leaf tea while it's still warm.

10. Dosage:

- Follow the suggested serving size stated on the tea box or the counsel of your healthcare physician or herbalist.

11. Consistency:

- For possible advantages, seek to take raspberry leaf tea regularly as instructed by your healthcare physician or herbalist. Consistency is necessary for herbal medicines to have an impact.

12. Monitor and Evaluate:

- Regularly check your PCOS symptoms and general well-being while utilizing raspberry leaf. Keep note of any modifications or upgrades. It may take some time to observe the results.

13. Professional Guidance:

- While raspberry leaf is usually regarded as safe, it's vital to include it in your PCOS treatment strategy under the advice of a healthcare physician or herbalist, particularly if you have underlying health concerns or are using drugs.

CHAPTER SIX

Herbs for Reducing Androgen Levels

Spearmint (Mentha spicata)

Spearmint (Mentha spicata) is a common herb that has been examined for its ability to help treat PCOS (Polycystic Ovary Syndrome) by lowering symptoms such as hirsutism (excessive hair growth) and hormonal abnormalities. If you use spearmint as part of your PCOS treatment strategy, you may make it as an herbal tea. Here's a broad guide on how to do so:

Ingredients and Equipment:

- Dried spearmint leaves (available in loose-leaf form or as tea bags)
- Water Honey or lemon (optional, for taste)

Instructions:

1. Choose High-Quality Spearmint Leaves:

- Look for high-quality dried spearmint leaves from a reliable vendor.
- You may get them in loose-leaf form or as pre-packaged tea bags.

2. Measure Spearmint Leaves:

- If using loose-leaf spearmint leaves, start with 1 to 2 tablespoons of dried leaves per cup of tea. You may modify the amount according to your preferences.
- If using tea bags, follow the suggested serving size on the label.

3. Boil Water:

- Boil a cup of Water using a kettle or on the stove. Make sure the Water is fresh and clean.

4. Preparing Spearmint Tea:

- Place the measured dried spearmint leaves in a cup.

5. Pour Boiling Water:

- Pour the boiling water over the spearmint leaves into the cup.
- Ensure that the leaves are thoroughly immersed.

6. Stir and Let It Steep:

- Use a spoon to whisk the spearmint leaves and hot Water together.
- Allow the spearmint leaves to soak in the boiling water for 5-10 minutes. This steeping period enables the tastes and therapeutic components to seep into the Water.

7. Strain (Optional):

- After steeping, you may filter the tea without the leaves if you like a transparent beverage. However, this step is optional.

8. Optional Flavoring:

- If desired, add honey or lemon to taste for flavour. These ingredients improve the flavour of the tea.

9. Cool and Enjoy:

- Allow the spearmint tea to cool to a comfortable drinking temperature.
- Enjoy the spearmint tea while it's still warm.

10. Dosage:

- Follow the suggested serving size stated on the tea box or the recommendation of your healthcare expert.

11. Consistency:

- For possible advantages in controlling PCOS symptoms, try sipping spearmint tea frequently. Some folks consume it every day.

12. Monitor and Evaluate:

- Regularly check your PCOS symptoms and general well-being while drinking spearmint tea. Keep note of any modifications or upgrades. Note that it may take some time to detect the results.

13. Professional Guidance:

- Spearmint tea is usually considered safe, but it's a good practice to include it in your PCOS treatment plan with the advice of a healthcare physician or trained dietitian, particularly if you have underlying health concerns or are taking medicines.

Spearmint tea is typically used as part of a comprehensive approach to PCOS treatment, which may include dietary changes, exercise, and other lifestyle adjustments.

Licorice Root (Glycyrrhiza glabra)

Licorice root (Glycyrrhiza glabra) may be used with care as a comprehensive approach to addressing PCOS (Polycystic Ovary Syndrome). Its primary ingredient, glycyrrhizin, has possible hormonal-balancing benefits. Still, it should be taken carefully and under the advice of a skilled healthcare physician or herbalist, owing to potential adverse effects when ingested in excess. Here's some essential advice on how to prepare and utilize liquorice root for a PCOS remedy:

- Liquorice root (dry liquorice root slices or liquorice root tea bags)
- Water Honey or lemon (optional, for taste)

Instructions:

1. Choose High-Quality Licorice Root:

- Look for high-quality dried liquorice root slices or tea bags from a trustworthy provider.

2. Measure Licorice Root:

- If using dried liquorice root slices, start with 1 to 2 pieces per cup of tea. You may modify the amount depending on your tastes and tolerance.
- If using liquorice root tea bags, follow the suggested serving size indicated on the label.

3. Boil Water:

- Boil a cup of Water using a kettle or on the stove. Ensure the Water is fresh and clean.

4. Preparing Licorice Root Tea:

- Place the measured liquorice root slices or tea bag in a cup.

5. Pour Boiling Water:

- Pour the boiling water over the liquorice root in the cup. Ensure that the source or tea bag is thoroughly immersed.

6. Stir and Let It Steep:

- Use a spoon to whisk the liquorice root and boiling Water together.
- Allow the liquorice root to soak in the boiling water for 5-10 minutes. This steeping period enables the beneficial chemicals to seep into the Water.

7. Strain (Optional):

- After steeping, you may drain the tea if you want a pure brew without the liquorice root or tea bag. However, this step is optional.

8. Optional Flavoring:

- If desired, add honey or lemon to taste for flavour.
- These ingredients enhance the flavour of the tea.

9. Cool and Enjoy:

- Allow the liquorice root tea to cool to a suitable drinking temperature.
- Enjoy the liquorice root tea while it's still warm.

10. Dosage:

- Follow the suggested serving size stated on the tea box or the counsel of your healthcare physician or herbalist.

11. Consistency:

- Take liquorice root tea frequently for possible advantages in treating PCOS symptoms, but be careful not to overconsume it.

12. Monitor and Evaluate:

- Regularly check your PCOS symptoms and general well-being while utilizing liquorice root. Keep note of any modifications or upgrades. Note that it may take some time to detect the results.

13. Professional Guidance:

- Liquorice root should be taken carefully and under a healthcare physician's or herbalist's advice, owing to possible adverse effects associated with excessive ingestion, including elevated blood pressure and potassium loss.

Liquorice root may be explored as part of a comprehensive PCOS treatment strategy, including dietary adjustments, exercise, and other lifestyle modifications.

Nettle Leaf (Urtica dioica)

Nettle leaf (Urtica dioica), popularly known as stinging nettle, is a herb historically utilized for its possible health advantages, including its high nutritional content and function in controlling numerous health disorders. Some persons with PCOS (Polycystic Ovary Syndrome) consider utilizing nettle leaves as part of their comprehensive care approach. Here's some essential advice on how to prepare and use nettle leaf for a PCOS remedy:

Ingredients and Equipment:

Dried nettle leaf (available in loose-leaf form or as tea bags) Water Honey or lemon (optional, for taste)

Instructions:

1. Choose High-Quality Nettle Leaf:

- Look for high-quality dried nettle leaf from a trusted vendor. You may get it in loose-leaf form or as pre-packaged tea bags.

2. Measure Nettle Leaf:

- Using loose-leaf nettle, start with 1 to 2 tablespoons of dried leaves per cup of tea. You may modify the amount according to your preferences.
- If using tea bags, follow the suggested serving size on the label.

3. Boil Water:

- Boil a cup of Water using a kettle or on the stove. Ensure the Water is fresh and clean.

4. Preparing Nettle Leaf Tea:

- Place the measured dried nettle leaf in a cup.

5. Pour Boiling Water:

- Pour the boiling water over the nettle leaf in the cup. Ensure that the leaves are thoroughly immersed.

6. Stir and Let It Steep:

- Use a spoon to whisk the nettle leaf and boiling Water together.

- Allow the nettle leaf to soak in the boiling water for 5-10 minutes. This steeping period enables the tastes and therapeutic components to seep into the Water.

7. Strain (Optional):

- After steeping, you may filter the tea if you want a pure beverage without the leaves or tea bag. However, this step is optional.

8. Optional Flavoring:

- If desired, add honey or lemon to taste for flavour. These ingredients improve the flavour of the tea.

9. Cool and Enjoy:

- Allow the nettle-leaf tea to cool to a suitable drinking temperature.

- Enjoy the nettle leaf tea while it's still warm.

10. Dosage:

- Follow the suggested serving size stated on the tea box or the counsel of your healthcare physician or herbalist.

11. Consistency:

- Try taking nettle leaf tea frequently for possible advantages in controlling PCOS symptoms. Some folks consume it every day.

12. Monitor and Evaluate:

- Regularly check your PCOS symptoms and general well-being while utilizing nettle leaf. Keep note of any modifications or upgrades. Note that it may take some time to detect the results.

13. Professional Guidance:

- Nettle leaf is typically considered safe for most individuals when ingested in moderation. However, it's a good practice to include it in your PCOS treatment plan with the advice of a healthcare physician or qualified dietitian, particularly if you have underlying health concerns or are taking drugs.

CHAPTER SEVEN

Holistic Approaches to PCOS Management

Combining Herbal Remedies with Diet and Exercise

Managing PCOS (Polycystic Ovary Syndrome) frequently takes a complex strategy, including herbal therapies, dietary adjustments, and regular exercise. Here's how you may adequately combine these aspects to help treat PCOS:

1. Herbal Remedies:

As noted before, herbal therapies such as chasteberry, spearmint, liquorice root, and nettle leaf might be regarded as supplementary treatments. However, it's vital to utilize them wisely and under the advice of a healthcare physician or herbalist.

2. Dietary Changes:

Adopting a PCOS-friendly diet may have a substantial influence on controlling the disease. Here are nutritional tips to consider:

- **Balanced Macronutrients:** Aim for balanced meals that contain carbs, proteins, and healthy fats to help stabilize blood sugar levels.

- **Low Glycemic Index (GI) Foods:** Choose foods with a low glycemic index to reduce blood sugar increases. This contains whole grains, veggies, and legumes.

- **Lean Protein Sources:** Incorporate lean protein sources such as chicken, fish, tofu, and lentils to maintain muscle health and balance blood sugar.

- **Fiber-Rich meals:** Include high-fibre meals, including fruits, vegetables, and whole grains, to assist with digestion and increase satiety.

- **Healthy Fats:** Consume sources of healthy fats, including avocados, nuts, seeds, and olive oil, to maintain hormonal balance.

- **Limit Sugary Foods and Beverages:** Reduce or eliminate sugary snacks and beverages to reduce insulin resistance.

- **Moderate Dairy:** Some persons with PCOS may benefit from limiting dairy intake or adopting dairy substitutes.

- **Portion Control:** Practice portion control to prevent overeating and maintain a healthy weight.

Exercise significantly controls PCOS by enhancing insulin sensitivity, supporting weight management, and lowering stress. Aim for aerobic workouts (e.g., brisk walking, cycling) and strength training exercises. Aim for at least 150 minutes of moderate-intensity aerobic exercise or 75 minutes of vigorous-intensity aerobic activity each week, combined with muscle-strengthening activities two or more days a week.

Beyond nutrition and exercise, consider these lifestyle changes:

- **Stress Management:** Practice stress-reduction practices such as mindfulness, yoga, meditation, or deep breathing exercises to assist in managing stress, which may increase PCOS symptoms.
- **Adequate Sleep:** Ensure you receive sufficient quality sleep since poor sleep patterns might impair hormone control.
- **Hydration:** Stay well-hydrated by drinking lots of Water throughout the day.
- **Regular Check-Ups:** Schedule frequent check-ups with your healthcare practitioner to monitor your

PCOS and modify your treatment strategy as required.

5. Healthcare Provider Guidance:

Work closely with a healthcare physician knowledgeable in treating PCOS to build a specific treatment strategy. They can help you choose the most suited herbal therapies, assess your Progress, and handle any unique health issues associated with PCOS.

6. Monitoring and Patience:

PCOS treatment may take time, and monitoring your symptoms and Progress is crucial. Be patient and make improvements to your strategy as required.

7. Individualized Approach:

PCOS affects everyone differently. Therefore, personalizing your treatment approach to your particular requirements and preferences is vital.

Remember that herbal therapies are one aspect of a complete PCOS management regimen. Diet, exercise, and lifestyle modifications are equally significant components.

Stress Reduction Techniques

Stress reduction approaches may be particularly effective for controlling PCOS (Polycystic Ovary Syndrome) since stress can increase PCOS symptoms and hormonal abnormalities. Here are various stress reduction tactics that you may implement into your everyday routine:

1. Mindfulness Meditation:

   Mindfulness meditation includes concentrating your attention on the current moment without judgment. Regular practice may help decrease stress and promote mental well-being. Various mindfulness meditation applications and guided sessions are accessible online to get you started.

2. Deep Breathing Exercises:

   Deep breathing techniques, such as diaphragmatic breathing or the 4-7-8 method, help trigger the body's relaxation response and decrease stress. These exercises are easy and can be done anywhere.

3. **Progressive Muscle Relaxation:**

Progressive muscle relaxation includes progressively tensing and relaxing distinct muscle groups to alleviate physical stress. It may help you become more aware of where you keep tension in your body and how to let go of it.

4. **Yoga:**

Yoga combines physical postures, breathing techniques, and mindfulness to relieve stress and promote relaxation. Regular yoga may increase flexibility, decrease muscular tension, and boost general well-being.

5. **Aromatherapy:**

Some essential oils, such as lavender, chamomile, and bergamot, offer relaxing qualities. You may use essential oils in a diffuser, as part of a bath, or for aromatherapy massage to help decrease stress.

6. **Regular Exercise:**

Exercise is not only excellent for physical health but also for stress reduction. It releases endorphins, which are natural mood boosters. Find a fitness regimen you love, whether walking, cycling, dancing or any other activity.

7. Social Support:

Sharing your problems and thoughts with friends, family, or a support group may give emotional support and lessen feelings of isolation, which can add to stress.

8. Healthy Diet:

A well-balanced diet with nutrient-rich meals may assist your body's stress response. Avoid excessive coffee and sugar, which may contribute to energy spikes and crashes, and prefer nutritious meals.

9. Time Management:

Effective time management helps lessen the stress associated with feeling overwhelmed by everyday chores. Make to-do lists, prioritize work, and establish reasonable objectives for yourself.

10. Quality Sleep:

Prioritize obtaining adequate restorative sleep. Establish a consistent sleep pattern and a pleasant sleep environment, and avoid electronics before night to increase the quality of your sleep.

11. Counselling or Therapy:

Speaking with a therapist or counsellor may equip you with skills and ways to manage stress and treat any underlying emotional problems that may lead to stress.

12. Hobbies & Relaxation Activities:

Engaging in hobbies and activities you like, such as reading, drawing, gardening, or listening to music, may bring a feeling of relaxation and happiness.

13. Limit Screen Time:

Excessive screen usage, particularly on social media, may add to stress. Consider establishing limits and taking frequent breaks from screens.

Remember that stress reduction is a personal process, and various strategies work for different individuals.

Mind-Body Practices for PCOS

Mind-body activities may be essential aids in controlling PCOS (Polycystic Ovary Syndrome) by increasing relaxation, lowering stress, and boosting general well-being. These practices concentrate on the relationship between the mind and body and may help you better manage your PCOS symptoms. Here are some mind-body techniques to consider:

a. **Yoga:** combines physical postures, breathing techniques, and awareness to relieve stress and promote relaxation. It may also increase flexibility, strength, and general fitness. Specific yoga positions, such as the "child's pose" and "butterfly pose," may be incredibly influential for PCOS by targeting the pelvic region.

b. **Tai Chi:** Tai Chi is a peaceful, low-impact martial art that stresses leisurely, flowing motions and deep breathing. It may assist in enhancing balance, decrease tension, and induce relaxation.

c. **Qi Gong:** Qi Gong is an ancient Chinese technique that incorporates gentle movements, breath control, and meditation to increase the flow of vital energy (qi) in the body. It may help relieve stress and enhance general well-being.

d. **Meditation:** Meditation includes concentrating on the present moment, relaxing the mind, and lowering tension. Mindfulness meditation may help you become more aware of your thoughts and emotions, helping you to handle stress more efficiently.

e. **Guided Imagery:** Guided imagery is utilizing your imagination to generate soothing mental pictures or situations. It may help alleviate stress and anxiety by redirecting your concentration away from stress.

f. **Breathing Exercises:** Deep breathing exercises, such as diaphragmatic breathing or the 4-7-8 method, help trigger the body's relaxation response and decrease stress. They are accessible practices that may be done anytime, anyplace.

g. **Biofeedback:** Biofeedback employs electronic monitoring to become aware of and regulate physiological processes such as heart rate and muscular tension. Learning to manage these processes may help decrease stress and enhance overall health.

h. **Progressive Muscle Relaxation:** This method includes progressively tensing and then releasing various muscle groups to alleviate physical stress. It may help you become more aware of where you keep tension in your body and how to let go of it.

i. **Hypnotherapy:** Hypnotherapy includes employing guided relaxation and focused concentration to treat particular difficulties, such as stress reduction or weight control. It may help transform unfavourable mental patterns and actions.

j. **Acupuncture:** Acupuncture is an ancient Chinese treatment that includes inserting tiny needles into particular spots on the body. Some people with PCOS find acupuncture helpful in controlling symptoms such as irregular periods and hormone abnormalities.

k. **Massage treatment:** Massage treatment may assist in alleviating muscular tension, enhance circulation, and promote relaxation. It might be particularly effective if you feel muscular pain or discomfort associated with PCOS.

l. **Mindful Eating:** Mindful eating entails paying great attention to the sensory experience of eating, such as the taste, texture, and smell of food. It may help you make better food choices and prevent emotional eating.

Finding mind-body activities that connect with you and fit into your lifestyle is crucial. Integrating these behaviours into your PCOS treatment strategy may improve overall well-being, stress, and symptom control.

CHAPTER EIGHT

Creating Personalized Herbal Regimens

Consultation with a Herbalist or Naturopath

Consulting with a herbalist or naturopath may be a helpful step in your effort to control PCOS (Polycystic Ovary Syndrome) with herbal therapies and natural techniques. These specialists may give specialized assistance, propose particular herbal treatments, and help you construct a holistic strategy suited to your unique circumstances. Here's what you may anticipate when meeting with a herbalist or naturopath for PCOS management:

1. Assessment and Evaluation:

> During your first session, the herbalist or naturopath will thoroughly assess your PCOS symptoms, medical history, dietary habits, lifestyle variables, and other pertinent information. They may ask questions about your menstrual cycle, hormone levels, stress levels, and general wellness.

2. Personalized Treatment Plan:

Based on the information acquired during the examination, the herbalist or naturopath will build a specific treatment plan for controlling your PCOS. This approach may include herbal medications, dietary advice, lifestyle improvements, and mind-body activities.

3. Herbal Recommendations:

The herbalist or naturopath will prescribe herbal medicines suited to your situation. They will explain how to prepare and use these herbs, the suggested dose, and any adverse effects or interactions with other drugs or supplements you may be taking.

4. Dietary Guidance:

Diet plays a vital part in controlling PCOS, and the herbalist or naturopath may give nutritional counselling customized to your requirements. They can help you design a balanced eating plan that promotes hormone balance and blood sugar management.

5. Lifestyle Recommendations:

Lifestyle adjustments may also be a crucial element in controlling PCOS. The herbalist or naturopath may advise stress reduction tactics, exercise routines, and other lifestyle adjustments to complement your treatment approach.

6. Follow-Up Appointments:

You will often have follow-up sessions with the herbalist or naturopath to assess your Progress, change your treatment plan as appropriate, and address any issues or questions.

7. Safety Precautions:

The herbalist or naturopath will emphasize your safety and well-being. They will address any possible hazards linked with herbal medicines and confirm that the selected therapies suit your unique health profile.

8. Collaboration with Healthcare Providers:

Your herbalist or naturopath must work with your primary healthcare practitioner or gynaecologist. This ensures that all parts of your PCOS therapy are coordinated and any possible interactions with drugs are examined.

9. Education and Empowerment:

Most of the meeting informs you about your problem and treatment choices. The herbalist or naturopath will enable you to take an active part in controlling your PCOS and making educated choices regarding your health.

When picking a herbalist or naturopath, search for licensed, qualified, and skilled practitioners in treating hormone imbalances, PCOS, or women's health. It's vital to speak honestly with them, ask questions, and discuss any concerns you may have regarding your PCOS treatment strategy. Integrating herbal medicines and natural techniques into your healthcare plan may be a valuable part of your path to better manage PCOS symptoms and enhance your overall well-being.

Building Your Herbal Medicine Cabinet

Building an herbal medicine cabinet for PCOS (Polycystic Ovary Syndrome) management entails choosing and stockpiling herbal treatments that may help relieve particular symptoms and support your general well-being. Here are some herbal choices you might explore for your PCOS herbal medication cabinet:

a. **Chasteberry (Vitex agnus-castus):** Chasteberry is widely used to manage menstrual cycles and hormonal abnormalities in PCOS. It may help reduce symptoms such as irregular periods and mood swings.

b. **Spearmint (Mentha spicata):** Spearmint tea or pills have anti-androgenic qualities, which may help decrease excessive hair growth (hirsutism) and hormonal abnormalities in PCOS.

c. **Licorice Root (Glycyrrhiza glabra):** Licorice root may help hormonal balance and promote adrenal function. It should be taken carefully owing to its possible adverse effects.

d. **Nettle Leaf (Urtica dioica):** Nettle leaf is rich in nutrients and may enhance general health. It may be suitable for lowering inflammation and supporting the body's systems.

e. **Cinnamon (Cinnamomum verum):** Cinnamon may help manage blood sugar levels, vital for treating insulin resistance in PCOS.

f. **Fenugreek (Trigonella foenum-graecum):** Fenugreek seeds may help manage blood sugar levels and enhance insulin sensitivity.

g. **Saw Palmetto (Serenoa repens):** Saw palmetto may aid in lowering hirsutism by preventing the activity of androgens (male hormones).

h. **Black Cohosh (Cimicifuga racemosa):** Black cohosh is occasionally used for its ability to treat menopausal symptoms and improve hormonal balance.

i. **Bitter Melon (Momordica charantia):** Bitter melon may help enhance insulin sensitivity and manage blood sugar levels.

j. **Dong Quai (Angelica sinensis):** Dong quai is a traditional Chinese herb renowned for improving hormonal balance and easing menstruation discomfort.

k. **White Peony (Paeonia lactiflora):** White peony may help regulate menstrual cycles and alleviate menstrual discomfort.

l. **Raspberry Leaf (Rubus idaeus):** Raspberry leaf is rich in nutrients and may help uterine health and hormonal balance.

m. **Sage (Salvia officinalis):** Sage tea may help decrease excessive perspiration and hot flashes, which some women with PCOS may experience.

n. **Milk Thistle (Silybum marianum):** Milk thistle enhances liver function, crucial for hormonal balance and cleansing.

When establishing your herbal medicine cabinet, keep the following points in mind:

- **Consultation:** Always speak with a healthcare physician or herbalist before adding herbal treatments to your regimen, particularly if you have underlying health concerns or are using drugs.

- **Quality:** Choose high-quality herbs from reliable suppliers to guarantee safety and efficacy.

- **Dosage:** Follow suggested doses supplied by healthcare experts or on the product label.

- **Safety:** Be careful of possible interactions and adverse effects of herbs, and quit usage if you develop unpleasant reactions.

- **Consistency:** Herbal treatments sometimes need persistent usage over time to realize possible effects.

- **Monitoring:** When using herbal medicines, keep track of your symptoms and general well-being.

- **Comprehensive Approach:** Remember that herbal medicines are only one aspect of a comprehensive PCOS management approach that may include diet, exercise, stress reduction, and other lifestyle improvements.

Your herbal medicine cabinet should suit your PCOS symptoms and requirements. Regular consultation with a healthcare physician or herbalist is crucial for efficient and safe PCOS treatment utilizing herbal therapies.

Keeping a PCOS Herbal Journal

Keeping a PCOS (Polycystic Ovary Syndrome) herbal notebook may be an excellent tool for monitoring your herbal medicines, symptoms, and general success. It helps you to monitor the effects of herbal therapies, spot trends, and make educated choices regarding your PCOS management. Here's how to develop and keep a PCOS herbal journal:

1. Choose a Journal Format:

You may use an actual notebook, a digital document, or a specialized journaling program on your computer or smartphone. Select a format that meets your tastes and is simple to access.

2. Create Sections or Categories:

Divide your diary into sections or categories to help you arrange material. Common portions may include:

- **Symptom Tracking:** Record PCOS-related symptoms such as irregular periods, hirsutism, mood swings, etc.

- **Herbal Remedies:** Document the herbal remedies you use, including the herb's name, dose, preparation technique, and frequency.

- **Diet and Lifestyle:** Note any dietary changes, exercise regimens, stress reduction measures, and lifestyle alterations.

- **Mood & Emotions:** Track your emotional well-being and stress levels.

- **Appointments & Consultations:** Record information from healthcare providers or herbalist visits.

- **Observations:** Use this part to write notable comments or experiences relating to your PCOS and herbal therapies.

3. Set a Regular Journaling Schedule:

Dedicate time to journaling frequently, whether daily, weekly, or as required. Consistency can help you spot patterns and analyze the efficacy of herbal medicines over time.

4. Record Details:

Be clear and thorough while making entries. Include dates, timings, and other pertinent information. For herbal medicines, record the name of the plant, preparation technique (e.g., tea, tincture), dose, and any adverse effects or changes in symptoms.

5. Monitor Symptoms:

Keep a careful watch on PCOS-related symptoms and how they evolve. This can help you judge if herbal medicines are making a difference.

Record your nutritional choices, exercise regimens, and stress reduction strategies. Note any changes in your behaviours and how they may influence your PCOS symptoms.

Regularly reread your diary entries to detect trends, improvements, or possible triggers. Look for links between herbal medicines, lifestyle modifications, and symptom changes.

Use your notebook to guide improvements to your PCOS treatment strategy. If you find patterns or specific treatments that appear incredibly successful or ineffective, share them with your healthcare professional or herbalist during your appointments.

Acknowledge and appreciate any changes in your PCOS symptoms or general well-being. Positive developments, even modest ones, are worth recognizing and appreciating.

Continue investigating and learning about PCOS and natural therapies. Use your journal to make notes of articles, books, or anything you encounter that may be related to your condition.

Remember that controlling PCOS is a journey, and your notebook is a helpful tool for monitoring your Progress and making educated choices regarding your health. Share your diary with your healthcare physician or herbalist during appointments to ensure your PCOS treatment strategy is personalized to your requirements and experiences.

www.ingramcontent.com/pod-product-compliance
Lightning Source LLC
Chambersburg PA
CBHW070819280726
48660CB00016B/2143